Paleo Bacon Cookbook

Lose Weight * Get Healthy * Eat Bacon

By Sasha Kendrick

Disclaimer

Table of Contents

Introduction

Paleolithic people never ate dairy, hardly ate cereal grains, and used only honey as a source of sugar. They got their carbohydrates and fiber from fruits and vegetables. They also ate meat from the animals they hunted, including the fat that provided them with a valuable energy source.

We may not hunt too many of the animals we eat these days, but we can still derive huge benefits from following a Paleo diet that supports the optimal functioning of our DNA.

And what's everyone's favorite meat and fat combo? Bacon, of course! With the embracing of meat and fat in the Paleo diet, bacon has become the "candy" of the Paleo world.

And so bacon lovers, not only can you have your bacon and eat it too, but you can also reap the laundry list of benefits from the Paleo diet by chewing down on your salty favorite.

*Paleo Bacon Cookbook: Lose Weight * Get Healthy * Eat Bacon* provides you with 30 bacon-licious recipes: six starters, six entrees, six side dishes, six desserts, and six treats. All including bacon, each recipe contains:

- serving size
- time involved
- equipment needed
- complete list of ingredients
- clear directions
- nutritional information

From scallops to chicken, chocolate to ice cream, you are sure to find bacon favorites in no time. And the best part? All of these recipes are strictly Paleo, to help you stick to your health and nutritional goals.

If you're new to the Paleo diet, included here is a brief, informative section on what the Paleo diet is, and how it is revolutionizing eating and overall health.

Bacon...Paleo...health... what's stopping you from taking a peek inside this wonderful book?

What is the Paleo Diet?

The Paleo diet operates from the premise that we have moved away from a diet that supports optimal functioning of our bodies.

This has lead to an explosion in rates of disease, obesity and a reliance on substances like sugar and caffeine to help us meet the demands of a 21st century lifestyle.

Advocates of the diet claim that we can reorder our bodies, keep it well-nourished and disease-free by eating a diet that resembles that of our hunter-gatherer ancestors.

The Paleo diet is a modern interpretation of that diet using real food ingredients and avoidance of processed, chemical-laden foods.

Foods to eat:

- Meat
- Fish
- Fowl
- Eggs
- Vegetables
- Fruits
- Nuts
- Seeds
- Healthy fats

Foods to avoid:

Grains

- Sugar
- Legumes
- Dairy
- Processed food
- Alcohol
- Starches
- Vegetable oils

What you eat; and, for some who take the basic principle further, how much you sleep, work, relax and play all fall under the Paleo banner.

We are learning more and more about how our current lifestyle makes us fat, sick, weak and miserable, and how important it is to make a radical change.

Starters

Broccoli Bacon Cashew Salad

Serves 4

Time involved: 5 minutes prepping; 15 minutes cooking

Equipment needed: 1 small pan; 1 frying pan; 1 large serving bowl

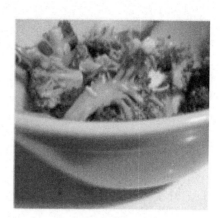

Ingredients

1 head of broccoli (cut into florets, stalk diced)
1/2 cup cashews
3 strips of bacon (diced)
1 tbsp olive oil

Directions

In water, boil broccoli on high heat for 5-7 minutes.

Discard water and place cooked broccoli in a large serving bowl.

In a frying pan, cook bacon for about 5 minutes, or until crispy.

Remove from pan and add to broccoli. Add in cashews and toss.

Nutrition Facts
Calories: 233; Fat: 18g; Carbs: 11g; Protein: 8g

Sweet Potato Bacon Muffins

Serves 4

Time involved: 10
minutes prepping;
45 minutes baking

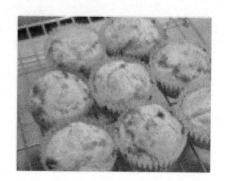

**Equipment
needed:** 1 grater; 1
mixing bowl; 1
muffin tray

Preheat oven to
400F°.

Ingredients

6 strips of bacon
1 large sweet potato
1 egg
1 1/2 tsp dried onion (minced)
1 bunch chives
1 tsp coconut oil
Sea salt to taste

Directions

Grate sweet potato and combine thoroughly with the
egg in a mixing bowl.

Grease muffin tray (4 muffins) with coconut oil.

Fold a strip of bacon inside each muffin slot to form a
cup shape.

Fill bacon-coated muffin tray with the sweet potato
mix.

Sprinkle in the onion, adding sea salt to taste.

Bake for 45 minutes.

Nutrition Facts
Calories: 160; Fat: 9g; Carbs: 12.5; Protein: 5g

Deviled Eggs with Bacon, Tuna, and Avocac

Serves 4

Time involved: 10 minutes prepping; 10 minutes cooking

Equipment needed: 1 bowl; 1 baking sheet

Preheat oven to 435F°.

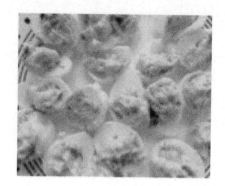

Ingredients

4 eggs (hard boiled, peeled)
1 small can tuna
1 avocado
1 tbsp extra virgin olive oil
Juice of 1/2 lemon
3 strips of bacon
Paprika and black pepper to taste

Directions

Lengthwise, cut eggs in half, and carefully scoop out the yolks into a bowl.

Put bacon in the oven and bake for 10 minutes.

Mash egg yolks with the avocado.

Then add tuna, black pepper, and lemon juice. Mix well.

Break bacon into little pieces and add to stuffing. Add in olive oil.

Scoop stuffing into the hollowed egg whites.

Nutrition Facts
Calories: 200; Fat: 13g; Carbs: 4g; Protein: 16g

Bacon Cream of Broccoli Soup

Serves 6

Time involved: 10 minutes prepping; 40 minutes cooking

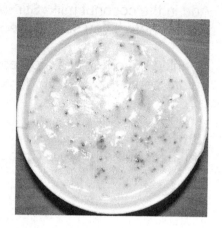

Equipment needed: 1 large pot; blender

Ingredients

1 head broccoli (chopped)
1 large onion (chopped)
2 tbsp coconut oil
2 garlic cloves (chopped finely)
2 stalks green onion (chopped)
1 quart chicken broth
2 tbsp ghee
Dash of cayenne and mustard power
1 cup coconut milk
4 strips of bacon (cooked, chopped)
Sprig of fresh parsley (chopped)
Sea salt and black pepper to taste

Directions

In a large pot, add onion and coconut oil on medium heat for 15 minutes.

Then add in green onion, garlic, broccoli, ghee, cayenne, mustard powder, salt and pepper, and broth. Allow to boil.

Covered, on medium-low heat, simmer for 20 minutes.

Turn off heat and use a blender to puree the mixture.

Add in the coconut milk. Stir. (Add salt and/or black pepper here if you so choose.)

Sprinkle bacon pieces atop each individual bowl before serving.

Nutrition Facts
Calories: 200; Fat: 19g; Carbs: 5.5g; Protein 4g

Garlic-Bacon Cabbage

Serves 4

Time involved: 10 minutes prepping; 30 minutes cooking

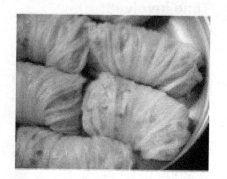

Equipment needed: aluminum foil; 1 sheet pan

Preheat oven to 425F°.

Ingredients

1 cabbage
4 strips of bacon (cooked, chopped)
4 cloves of garlic
4 tsp olive oil

Directions

Cut cabbage into quarters.

On each piece of cabbage, sprinkle garlic, olive oil, and cooked bacon.

Separately wrap in aluminum foil.

Cook in oven for 25-30 minutes.

Nutrition Facts
Calories: 150; Fat: 14g; Carbs: 2g; Protein: 4.5g

Avocado Bacon Dip

Serves 3

Time involved: 10-15 minutes total

Equipment needed: 1 skillet; 1 mixing bowl

Ingredients

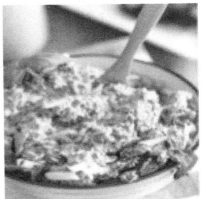

3 strips of smoked bacon
1 avocado
1 clove of garlic (minced)
1 tsp chives (sliced finely)
1/2 tomato (diced)
Sea salt and black pepper (to taste)

Directions

In a skillet, cook the bacon until crispy and browned. Let cool, and chop up the bacon into ½ inch pieces.

Peel and remove pit from avocado. In a mixing bowl, mash until smooth.

Stir in the garlic, tomato, and chives. Add sea salt and black pepper to taste.

Add in bacon pieces and mix well.

Nutrition Facts

Calories: 140; Fat: 13g; Carbs: 4g; Protein: 3g

Entrees

Honey-Mustard, Bacon-Wrapped Chicken

Serves 8

Time involved: 15 minutes prepping; 45 minutes baking

Equipment needed: 1 mallet; 1 mixing bowl; 1 brush; 1 baking pan

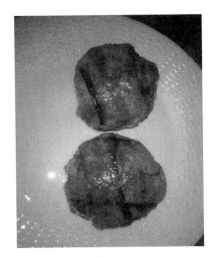

Preheat oven to 400F°.

Ingredients

8 boneless chicken breast halves
8 strips bacon
4 tbsp honey
3 tbsp mustard
2 jalapeños

Directions

Flatten chicken to 1/2 inch thickness with mallet.

Slice jalapeños in fourths, removing all seeds.

Roll one piece of jalapeño inside each chicken half.

Stir honey and mustard together in a bowl until smooth.

Spread honey-mustard mix on each piece of chicken.

Wrap each piece of chicken in one strip of bacon.

Place in a baking pan and bake for 35-45 minutes.

Nutrition Facts
Calories: 210; Fat: 10g; Carbs: 5g; Protein: 24g

Bacon Sea Scallops

Serves 4

Time involved:
10 minutes
prepping; 20-25
minutes cooking

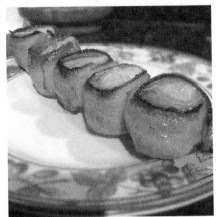

**Equipment
needed:** 1 skillet

Ingredients

1/2 lb bacon
12 sea scallops
3 shallots
(chopped)
5 kale leaves
1 tbsp chives
(fresh, chopped)
1 tbsp basil (fresh, chopped)

Directions

Chop bacon into small pieces. Cook in a skillet on over medium heat for 5-7 minutes.

Add in shallots and sauté for another 5 minutes.

Remove mixture and set aside.

In the same skillet, add scallops, and cook for 5 minutes in the bacon fat.

Add in the bacon mixture, basil, chives, and kale leaves with the scallops.

Cook for another 3 minutes, stirring.

Serve!

Nutrition Facts
Calories: 375; Fat: 24g; Carbs: 3g; Protein: 34g

Bacon Maple Brussels Sprouts

Serves 4

Time involved:
10 minutes prepping; 30 minutes baking/cooking

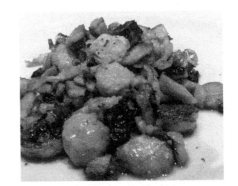

Equipment needed: 1 roasting pan; 1 skillet; 1 mixing bowl

Preheat oven to 350F°.

Ingredients

1 lb Brussels sprouts
4 strips of bacon
1 tbsp bacon fat
1 Granny Smith apple
2/3 cups almonds (slivered)
2 tsp maple vinegar
1/4 tsp sea salt

Directions

Cut the bases off of the Brussels sprouts. Cut each sprout in half.

Coat each Brussels sprout half in bacon fat and evenly spread out in a roasting pan.

Let roast for 20 minutes, or until soft on the inside and a little crispy on the outside.

In a skillet, cook bacon over medium heat until crispy.

Remove from heat, let dry on a paper towel, and then chop finely until crumbled.

Core the Granny Smith apple.

Dice, then mix with bacon in a bowl.

Chop the slivered almonds into finer pieces, then add to apple and bacon bowl.

Move the Brussels sprouts to the bowl.

Sprinkle with 2 tsp of maple vinegar and 1/4 tsp of salt. Mix thoroughly, and serve warm.

Nutrition Facts
Calories: 165; Fat: 8g; Carbs: 20g; Protein: 7g

Bacon-Wrapped Pork Tenderloin Skewers

Serves 4

Time involved: 15 minutes prepping; 10 minutes grilling

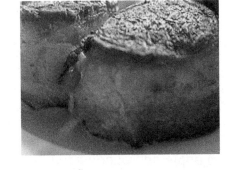

Equipment needed: food processor; skewers; 1 brush

Ingredients

2 pork tenderloins (about 1 lb each)
Bacon strips (will need one strip per chunk of pork)
2 cups fresh parsley
4 cloves of garlic
1/2 tsp black pepper
1/2 tsp red pepper flakes
1/4 tsp sea salt
1/4 cup white wine vinegar
1/2 cup extra virgin olive oil
2 tbsp water

Directions

In a food processor, pulse black pepper, pepper flakes, salt, parsley, and garlic.

Add white vinegar and water. Blend.

Carefully pour in olive oil while blending.

Set sauce aside!
Slice tenderloins into 2 inch thick chunks.

Wrap one strip of bacon around each chunk of tenderloin.

Skewer 3-4 chunks together. Spread some of the sauce over each chunk of bacon-wrapped tenderloin.

Grill over medium-high heat for about 4 minutes each side, brushing more sauce as you flip.

Serve with extra sauce.

Nutrition Facts
Calories: 385; Fat: 40g; Carbs: 3g; Protein: 7g

Squash and Bacon Frittata

Serves 4

Time involved: 5
minutes prepping;
25-30 minutes
cooking

**Equipment
needed:** 1 good-
sized skillet; 1
mixing bowl; 1
whisk

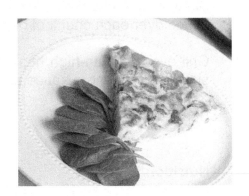

Preheat oven to
375F°.

Ingredients

6 strips of bacon (diced)
1/2 red bell pepper (diced)
1/2 yellow onion (diced)
1 yellow squash (diced)
1/2 cup sun-dried tomatoes (diced)
8 eggs
1/4 tsp dried dill
1 tbsp dried oregano
Sea salt and black pepper to taste

Directions

Over medium heat, add bacon to a good-sized skillet
and cook for 3 minutes.

Then add onion and continue cooking for another 3
minutes.

Add in squash, bell pepper, and sun-dried tomatoes. Cook for 5 minutes.

In a mixing bowl, whisk eggs with oregano, dill, salt, and pepper.

Add egg mixture to the skillet and cook for about 15 minutes, or until eggs are cooked through the middle.

Let cool slightly. Slice and serve.

Nutrition Facts
Calories: 300; Fat: 22g; Carbs: 5g; Protein 18g

Balsamic Jam-Topped Bacon Burgers

Serves 3

Time involved:
10 minutes prepping; 20-25 minutes cooking

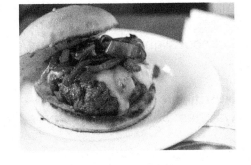

Equipment needed: 1 saucepan; grill; 1 mixing bowl

Jam Ingredients

4 strips of bacon
(chopped into ½" pieces)
1 red onion (sliced thinly)
1/3 cup balsamic vinegar
1/2 tsp Dijon mustard
1/3 cup water
Sea salt and black pepper (to taste)

Burger Ingredients

2 strips of bacon (minced)
1 lb ground beef
Worcestershire sauce (a healthy dash)
Sea salt and black pepper (to taste

Jam Directions

Over medium heat, cook bacon until lightly browned in a sauce pan.

Remove bacon and place on a paper towel.

Using the bacon grease in the same pan, add in onion and season with sea salt and black pepper. Cover the pan for two minutes.

Uncover the pan, add in a splash of water, and let cook until onions are soft and browned.

Mix in the balsamic vinegar, Dijon mustard, and remainder of the water.

Put the bacon back in the pan, bringing the mixture to a simmer.

Once thickened, remove from heat and set aside.

Burger Directions

Add ground beef, Worcestershire sauce, and a healthy pinch of sea salt and black pepper to a mixing bowl.

Mix well and form into patties (should make three).

Grill each burger for about five minutes on each side, or until cooked to your liking.

Serve with jam on top.

Nutrition Facts
Calories: 385; Fat: 20g; Carbs: 4g; Protein: 41g

Side Dishes

Bacon-Topped Broccoli and Cauliflower Chowder

Serves 8

Time involved: 5-7 minutes prepping; 20 minutes cooking

Equipment needed: blender; 1 large saucepan

Ingredients

4 cups broccoli (chopped, steamed)
4 cups cauliflower (chopped, steamed)
2 cups chicken or beef broth
5 gloves of garlic (roasted)
4 strips of bacon (chopped, baked)
Sea salt and black pepper to taste

Directions

Use a blender to blend the broccoli with 1 cup of the broth.

Add in cauliflower with the other cup of broth and mix together until smooth.

Add roasted garlic and blend again until smooth.

Over medium heat, put in the puree mixture in a sauce pan.

Add in sea salt and black pepper to taste.

Let simmer for 10 minutes, stirring occasionally.

Add more broth (1/4 cup at a time) if soup is too thick.

Garnish with chopped bacon.

Nutrition Facts
Calories: 80; Fat: 1.3 g; Carbs: 5.5g; Protein: 12.5

Bacon-Wrapped Pineapple and Pecan Dates

Makes 12

Time involved: 10-15 minutes prepping; 20-30 minutes baking

Equipment needed: toothpicks; 1 baking sheet

Preheat oven to 425F°.

Ingredients

2 dozen pecans (halved)
12 dried dates
12 strips bacon
1-2 cups fresh pineapple
(should be enough to make 12, 1 inch chunks)

Directions

Slice the dates lengthwise and remove all the pits.

Put two pecan halves in the center of each date to replace the pit.

Slice bacon in half (approx. 4 inches for each half)

Wrap one piece of bacon around each pecan-stuffed date. Fasten with a toothpick.

Wrap the leftover bacon pieces around each chunk of pineapple and fasten with a toothpick.

Place both the bacon-wrapped dates and pineapple on a baking sheet.

Bake for 20-30 minutes, or until bacon is cooked to your preference

Nutrition Facts
Calories: 140; Fat: 8g; Carbs: 10g; Protein 7g

Bacon and Onion Asparagus

Serves 4

Time involved: 5 minutes prepping; 15 minutes cooking

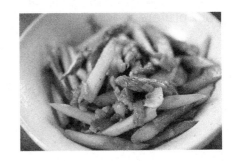

Equipment needed: 1 skillet; serving dish

Ingredients

1 bunch fresh asparagus (about 20 stalks)
4 strips bacon (sliced)
2 oz yellow onion (sliced)
Sea salt and black pepper to taste

Directions

Break off the bottoms (about 1/2 inch) of each asparagus stalk. Cut into 2 inch pieces.

In a skillet over medium heat, brown the bacon.

Remove from heat and set aside on a paper towel.

In the same skillet, with bacon grease, add in the onion until it begins to brown.

Then add in the pieces of asparagus, and sauté for 2-3 minutes.

Pour mixture in a serving dish and top with bacon pieces.

Nutritional Information
Calories: 100; Fat: 7g; Carbs: 5g; Protein: 5g

Cauliflower with Bacon and Leek

Serves 6-8

Time involved:
5 minutes prepping; 20 minutes cooking

Equipment needed: grater or food processor; 1 large skillet

Ingredients

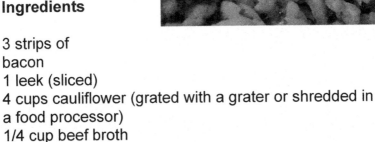

3 strips of bacon
1 leek (sliced)
4 cups cauliflower (grated with a grater or shredded in a food processor)
1/4 cup beef broth
Black pepper and sea salt to taste

Directions

Cut bacon into small pieces. In a large skillet over medium heat, fry bacon. Set aside, leaving bacon grease in the skillet.

Over medium heat, cook leek in bacon grease until soft.

Add in cauliflower and cook until soft. Stir regularly.

Add black pepper and/or sea salt to taste.

Then add broth, stir, and cover, lowering heat to medium-low.

Cook for 5 minutes, occasionally stirring.

Remove cover. Add bacon into the mix and stir together.

Nutrition Facts
Calories: 70; Fat: 4g; Carbs: 5g; Protein: 3g

Butternut Bacon Squash with Greens

Serves 12

Time involved: 5-10 minutes prepping; 20 minutes cooking

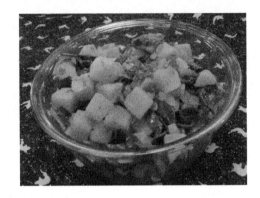

Equipment needed: peeler; 1 large pan; 1 skillet

Ingredients

1 lb bacon (diced)
1 butternut squash (peeled, seeded, and cubed)
1 zucchini (diced)
1 bunch chard (diced)
1 tsp olive oil
1 tsp balsamic vinegar

Directions

Place cubed butternut squash in a large pan and cover with water.

Boil for 5-7 minutes, or until squash is tender.

While squash boils: Cook bacon in a skillet until browned.

Drain the squash and add to the skillet with the bacon, also adding in the chard and zucchini.

Pour the olive oil and balsamic vinegar over mixture, toss, and serve.

Nutrition Facts
Calories: 210; Fat: 16g; Carbs: 2.5g; Protein: 14g

Bacon, Lettuce, and Pesto Salad

Serves 4

Time involved: 15 minutes total

Equipment needed: 1 mixing bowl; food processor; 1 large frying pan

Ingredients

3 tomatoes (chopped)
1 green onion (sliced)
12 strips of bacon
3 garlic cloves
1 tsp sea salt
1 cup cashews
1 bunch cilantro
1 tbsp olive oil

Directions

Add sliced green onion and chopped tomatoes into a mixing bowl. Set aside.

Over medium heat, add bacon to a large frying pan, and cook for 2-3 minutes, flipping the bacon.

Once cooked, place bacon on paper towels to absorb some grease

While bacon cooks: Put garlic, sea salt, cashews, and the cilantro in a food processor.

When cashews become finely chopped, drizzle in the olive oil as the processor continues to run. Keep running until pesto is at a consistency of your liking.

Chop up 10 strips of bacon and add to the tomato and onion mixture in your mixing bowl. Set the last 2 strips of bacon aside.

Then add the pesto into your mixing bowl, and stir together thoroughly.

Transfer the completed Pesto Salad into a serving bowl, garnishing with the two remaining strips of bacon.

Nutrition Facts
Calories: 250; Fat: 4 g; Carbs: 16g; Protein: 6g

Desserts

Maple Bacon Doughnuts

Makes 6-8

Time involved:
10-20 minutes
prepping; 20-25
minutes baking

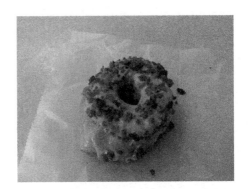

**Equipment
needed:**
doughnut pan; 2
mixing bowls;
blender; cooling
rack

Preheat oven to 350F°.

Doughnut Ingredients

4 eggs
1 3/4 cups almond flour
2 tbsp coconut flour
1 tbsp baking soda
1/2 cup maple syrup
1/4 cup coconut oil (melted)
1 tsp cinnamon
1 tsp vanilla extract
1/3 cup bacon (crumbled)

Glaze Ingredients

1/4 cup coconut butter
1/4 cup coconut milk
1/4 cup maple syrup

3 tbsp honey
2 tbsp + 1 tsp shortening
6 strips bacon (crumbled for topping)

Doughnut Directions

Grease donut pan.

Mix almond flour, coconut flour, baking soda, and cinnamon in a medium bowl.

Mix eggs, maple syrup, coconut oil, and vanilla extract in a separate bowl.

Mix in bacon crumbles. Stir.

Carefully pour the batter into the doughnut pan, filling each mold about 2/3 full.

Bake for 20 minutes, or until toothpick comes out clean.

Allow to cool on cooling rack.

Glaze Directions

Combine all ingredients in a blender until smooth, but thick.

Making sure the doughnuts have completely cooled, dip one side of each donut in the glaze and return to the cooling rack.

Top with bacon crumbles.

Nutrition Facts
Calories: 330; Fat: 19g; Carbs: 31g; Protein 9g

Bacon Truffles

Makes 10

Time involved:
10-15 minutes
total

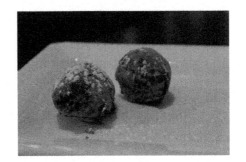

**Equipment
needed:** food
processor;
cookie sheet

Ingredients

1/2 cup dates
(pitted, chopped)
6 strips bacon (cooked)
1/4 tsp sea salt
2 tbsp cocoa powder
1 tbsp bacon grease

Directions

Mix dates, bacon, sea salt, cocoa powder, and bacon grease in a food processor until mixture is soft and smooth.

Form into 1 inch balls and place on a cookie sheet.

Place cookie sheet in the freezer for about an hour.

Enjoy!

Nutrition Facts
Calories: 90; Fat: 2g; Carbs: 7g; Protein: 4g

Bacon Cookies

Makes 30

Time involved: 10 minutes prepping; 35-40 minutes baking

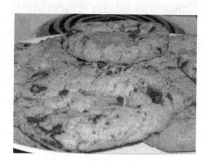

Equipment needed: 2 mixing bowls; 1 baking sheet; parchment paper; beater

Preheat oven to 350F°.

Ingredients

1 tsp baking soda
1 tsp sea salt
1 tsp vanilla extract
1 1/2 cup semisweet chocolate chips
1/2 cup coconut oil
3/4 cup maple syrup
2 eggs
3 cups almond flour
5 strips bacon (raw)

Directions

Toss bacon in 1/4 cup of maple syrup in a mixing bowl.

Place bacon on a baking sheet lined with parchment paper. Bake bacon for 20 minutes.

Remove bacon from oven and let cool. Crumble for the cookie batter.

Heat oven to 375F°.

Combine all dry ingredients in a mixing bowl.

In a smaller mixing bowl, beat eggs, 1/2 cup maple syrup, and vanilla extract.

Then pour mixture in with the dry ingredients and beat until full combined. Mix in candied bacon and chocolate chips and stir.

Form balls (about tbsp size) of dough on a baking sheet with parchment paper.

Bake cookies for 15 minutes.

Nutrition Facts
Calories: 130; Fat: 9g; Carbs: 13g; Protein: 2g

Bacon Maple Ice Cream

Serves 3

Time involved: 20 minutes total

Equipment needed: aluminum foil; 1 baking sheet; blender; ice cream maker

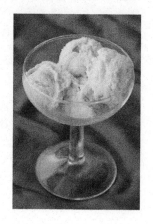

Preheat oven to 350F°.

Ingredients

1 can coconut milk
1/3 cup maple syrup
3 strips bacon
1 tsp vanilla extract

Directions

Lay bacon strips on aluminum foil in a baking sheet.

Cook until crispy enough to crumble.

Once bacon is finished, put coconut milk, maple syrup, and vanilla extract in a blender.

Mix well.

Place your ice cream maker bowl on your ice cream maker and start it.

Pour ingredients through the top.

After about 5 minutes, or when ice cream starts to solidify, add in bacon crumbles.

Make sure bacon mixes in well.

Put ice cream in a bowl and set in freezer to your liking.

Nutrition Facts
Calories: 200; Fat: 8g; Carbs: 24g; Protein: 7g

Maple-Pecan Bacon Bars

Makes 8

Time involved:
25 minutes
prepping; 40
minutes
baking/cooking

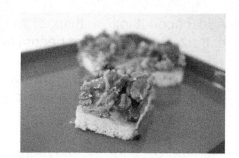

**Equipment
needed:** food
processor; 1
mixing bowl; 1
small baking dish;
1 large skillet

Preheat oven to 375F°.

Ingredients

2 1/4 cups pecans (unsalted)
3/4 cup almond flour
1/4 cup coconut oil (melted)
3 pear halves (canned)
3 dates (pitted, soaked in hot water for 15 minutes)
2 strips bacon (cubed)
1 egg (beaten)
4 tbsp maple syrup
1 tsp vanilla extract
1/2 tsp baking soda
1/2 tsp baking powder
Sea salt
Coconut oil spray

Directions

In a food processor, add 1 1/2 cups of almonds and process until fine.

Add coconut oil, 1 tbsp of maple syrup, and vanilla extract. Process until it becomes a batter.

Pour batter into a mixing bowl and add almond flour, baking soda, baking powder, a sprinkle of salt, and the egg. Stir to mix.

With the coconut oil spray, grease a small baking dish.

Evenly pour batter into baking dish. Bake for 20 minutes.

While batter bakes: Place pears and dates in the food processor and process until pureed. Remove and set aside.

Remove baked batter from the oven (the base layer of the bars) and spoon the pear and date puree evenly over the layer.

Place back in the oven for another 10 minutes, then take out and set aside.

In a large skillet over medium heat, place bacon cubes. Cook until very crispy, almost like bacon bits.

Add remaining 3/4 cup of pecans to food processor until roughly chopped, and set aside.

When bacon is done, remove from skillet, but leave skillet on the stove top.

Add in the pecans and toast until warm.

Add bacon back in the pan and stir together.

Remove skillet from heat and add the remaining 3 tbsp of maple syrup. Stir well to combine.

Evenly spoon the pecan-bacon mixture over the cooked bars.

Allow to cool fully, for it will become very sticky.

Nutrition Facts
Calories: 340; Fat: 31g; Carbs: 14g; Protein: 5g

Chocolate Bacon Cupcakes with Dark Chocolate Frosting

Makes 8-9

Time involved: 10 minutes prepping; 40 minutes cooking

Equipment needed: skillet; large mixing bowl; small mixing bowl; cupcake tins or silicone moulds; saucepan

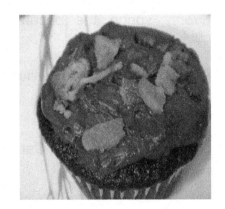

Preheat oven to 350F°.

Cupcake Ingredients

4 strips bacon (cut into 1/2 in. pieces)
2 cups almond flour
1/2 tsp sea salt
1/4 cup unsweetened cocoa powder
1/2 tsp baking soda
1/2 cup maple syrup
2 eggs (large)
1 tbsp vanilla extract

Dark Chocolate Frosting Ingredients

1/2 cup of 100% cacao dark chocolate
1/3 cup maple syrup
Pinch of sea salt
1/2 tbsp coconut milk
Directions

Cook bacon until halfway cooked (still pretty fatty) in a large skillet.

While bacon cooks: Mix all dry ingredients -- almond flour, cocoa powder, sea salt, and baking soda -- in a large mixing bowl.

In a smaller mixing bowl, combine eggs, vanilla extract, and maple syrup. Let it sit for 5 minutes.

Combine wet mix and dry mix until blended together.

Spoon batter into cupcake tins about 3/4 of the way full.

Bake for 12-15 minutes.

Let cool for 15 minutes on a cooling rack.

Frosting:
In a small saucepan, combine all ingredients over low heat.

Stir frequently until chocolate is melted, or for about 8-10 minutes.

Let cool for 10 minutes, and then spoon a small amount atop each cupcake.

Nutrition Facts
Calories: 150; Fat: 5g; Carbs: 21g; Protein: 5g

Treats

Bacon Nutty Bar

Makes 10

Time involved: 10-15 minutes total

Equipment needed: double-broiler or microwave; 1 cookie sheet; parchment paper

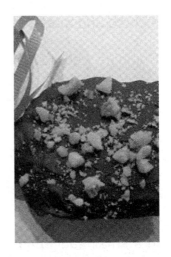

Ingredients

1 cup dark chocolate chips
1 tsp coconut oil
1/4 cup toasted walnuts (or any nut of your preference)
4 strips bacon (chopped, cooked)
1/2 tsp sea salt

Directions

Melt chocolate chips with coconut oil over low heat in a double-broiler, or in the microwave for 30 seconds.

Stir vigorously. (If not melted through, place in microwave for only 10 seconds at a time to avoid burning the chocolate.)

Over a cookie sheet, spread the melted chocolate on parchment paper. Set aside to cool.

When chocolate hasn't yet completely hardened, sprinkle the walnuts, sea salt, and bacon evenly over the top.

Roughly chop before serving.

Nutrition Facts
Calories: 120; Fat: 9g; Carbs: 8g; Protein: 4g

Flourless Bacon-Mocha Brownies

Makes 12

Time involved: 10 minutes prepping; 30 minutes baking

Equipment needed: 1 mixing bowl; whisk; 9x9 inch pan; parchment paper

Preheat oven to 375F°.

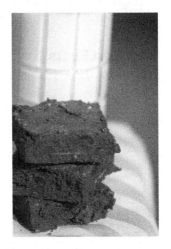

Ingredients

4 oz dark chocolate (melted and cooled)
1/2 cup coconut oil (melted and cooled)
1/2 cup maple syrup
3 eggs
1/2 cup + 2 tbsp unsweetened cocoa powder
2 tbsp coffee (the stronger the better)
2 tbsp finely ground coffee
2 strips bacon (chopped)

Directions

Combine the dark chocolate, coconut oil, maple syrup, and eggs in a mixing bowl.

Over the wet ingredients, carefully sift the cocoa powder. Whisk evenly.

Add coffee and coffee grinds and stir well.

Place a piece of parchment paper in a 9x9 inch pan, and fill with brownie batter.

Top with bacon pieces, and bake for 30 minutes.

Sprinkle with sifted cocoa powder for garnish.

Nutrition Facts
Calories: 196; Fat: 14g; Carbs: 15g; Protein: 3g

Egg Muffins with Bacon

Makes 12

Time involved: 10 minutes prepping; 15-20 minutes baking

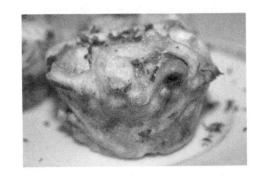

Equipment needed: 1 skillet; 1 muffin tin (12 muffin spaces); 1 mixing bowl

Preheat oven to 350F°.

Ingredients

6 eggs
3 tbsp coconut oil
1 cup mushrooms (chopped)
1 cup spinach (chopped)
4 strips bacon (cooked, chopped)
2 bunches of chives (chopped)
1/4 cup onion (chopped)

Directions

Heat 1 tbsp coconut oil in a skillet.

Sauté onions and mushrooms in the skillet until brown.

Lightly spread 1 tbsp coconut oil over muffin tin. (12 muffins)

In a bowl, scramble eggs. Add chives, bacon, mushrooms, and onions.

Separate mixture into muffin tins.

Bake for 15-20 minutes.

Nutrition Facts
Calories: 100; Fat: 8g; Carbs: .8g; Protein: 5g

Berry Bacon Bites with Dairy-Free Chocolate Sauce

Makes 12

Time involved: 10 minutes prepping; 10-12 minutes baking

Equipment needed: 1 baking tray; parchment paper; toothpicks; fork

Preheat oven to 450F°.

Berry Ingredients

24 medium-sized strawberries
12 strips of bacon
Black pepper to taste

Sauce Ingredients

1/2 cup coconut milk (full fat)
4 oz dark chocolate chips

Berry Directions

Line a baking tray with parchment paper.

Trim tops of strawberries.

Cut bacon strips in half, and wrap around each strawberry. The end of the bacon strip should overlap around the strawberry.

Secure with a toothpick and place strawberries, trimmed-side down, on the baking tray. Season with black pepper

Cook for 10-12 minutes, or until the edges of the bacon has begun to brown.

Remove and place each individual bacon-wrapped strawberry on paper towels to absorb excess grease.

Sauce Directions

Heat coconut milk until hot in the microwave or on the stovetop.

Using a fork, stir the chocolate chips in with the coconut milk until completely melted

Serve strawberries warm or cold.

Nutrition Facts
Calories: 175; Fat: 14g; Carbs: 9g; Protein: 5g

Bacon Zucchini Bites

Makes 6

Time involved: 10 minutes prepping; 25 minutes baking

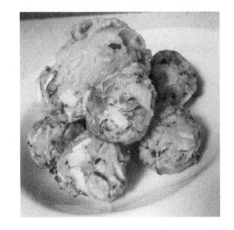

Equipment needed: 1 mixing bowl; 1 baking tray; parchment paper

Preheat oven to 400F°.

Ingredients

2 medium zucchinis (grated)
1 onion (chopped finely)
2 strips of bacon (diced)
2 eggs (beaten lightly)
1/4 cup coconut flour
1/2 tsp cumin
1 tsp paprika
Sea salt and black pepper to taste

Directions

In a bowl, mix zucchini, onion, and bacon.

Add in eggs and combine.

Sift in coconut flour and stir.

Add in cumin, paprika, salt, and pepper. Mix well.
Mold spoonfuls of mixture into bite-size balls.

Place the balls on a baking tray lined with parchment paper, and cook in the oven for 25 minutes.

Nutrition Facts
Calories: 40; Fat: 2g; Carbs: 4g; Protein 3g

Bacon Almond Butter Cookies

Makes 12-14

Time involved: 5-10 minutes prepping; 10 minutes baking

Equipment needed: 1 mixing bowl; 1 cookie sheet; mixer or beater

Preheat oven to 350F°.

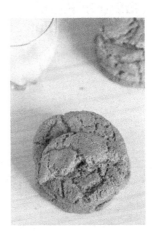

Ingredients

6 strips of bacon (cooked and chopped)
1 cup almond butter
1 cup coconut palm sugar
1 egg
1 tbsp baking soda
 Dash of sea salt

Directions

Using a mixer (or beaters), blend the almond butter and coconut palm sugar together.

Add in the egg and baking soda.

Fold in the bacon and add a dash of sea salt. Mix well.

On a cookie sheet, place tablespoon-sized balls of dough.

Bake for 10 minutes, then let cool before eating.
Nutrition Facts

Calories: 150; Fat: 36g; Carbs: 3g; Protein: 6g

Conclusion

Embracing the Paleo diet reaps long-term health benefits. Former research biochemist and author of *The Paleo Solution -- The Original Human Diet*, Robb Wolf, says that the Paleo diet is the healthiest way to eat because "it works with your genetics to help you stay lean, strong and energetic."

Unlike today's modern diet of refined food, sugar, and trans fat, the Paleo Diet incorporates only lean proteins, fruits and vegetables, and healthy fats from seeds, nuts, fish oil, and olive oil.

Although it might seem restrictive, there is plenty of delicious variety involved in Paleo meals, snacks, and desserts -- especially when you add in your favorite bacon!

With 30 recipes -- six starters, six entrees, six side dishes, six desserts, and six treats -- *Paleo Bacon Cookbook: Lose Weight * Get Healthy * Eat Bacon* offers tasty bacon options to suit your Paleo Diet needs.

Including serving size, time involved, equipment needed, a thorough list of ingredients, clear directions, and practical nutritional information for each recipe, this bacon compilation offers options that will certainly suit your taste buds *and* your Paleo diet needs.

Other Books by Sasha Kendrick

25 Days of Paleo Christmas Cookies and Other Holiday Indulgences: Your 25-Day Step-By-Step Guide to Creating Guilt-Free, Gluten-Free Sweets and Treats with Recipes Your Friends Will Be Begging For

*Paleo Bacon Cookbook: Lose Weight * Get Healthy * Eat Bacon*

Paleo Cravings: Your Favorite Comfort Foods Made Paleo

Paleo Easter Cookbook: Fast and Easy Recipes for Busy Moms

Paleo Party Food Cookbook: Make Your Friends Love You With Delicious & Healthy Party Food!

Paleo Pizza Cookbook: Lose Weight and Get Healthy by Eating the Food You Love

Paleo Valentine's Day Cookbook: Quick, Easy Recipes That Will Melt Your Lover's Heart
Simple Easy Paleo: Fast Fabulous Paleo Recipes with 5 Ingredients or Less

Other Books in the Paleo Kitchen and Health Series

Coconut Health Made Simple: Coconut Oil Cures & Health Hacks to Lose Weight, Lower Cholesterol, Improve Your Memory, Hair, & Skin

Break Free From Emotional Eating: Stop Overeating and Start Losing Weight

* * *

Available on Kindle and in paperback.

Books by Green Hills Press

Movie and TV Books in the British Drama series

Call The Midwife!: Your Backstage Pass to the Era and the Making of the PBS TV Series

Doctor Who: 200 Facts on the Characters and Making of the BBC TV Series

Downton Abbey: Your Backstage Pass to the Era and Making of the TV Series

Mr Selfridge: Your Backstage Pass to the True Harry Selfridge Story and Making of the PBS TV Series

Pride & Prejudice: Your Backstage Pass to Jane Austen's Novel and The Making of the BBC TV Series, Starring Colin Firth

Sherlock Lives! 100+ Facts on Sherlock and the Smash Hit BBC TV Series

The Bletchley Park Enigma: 200+ Facts on the Story of Alan Turing That Inspired The Smash Hit Movie "The Imitation Game" Starring Benedict Cumberbatch

Books in the Royals and Celebrities series

KATE: Loyal Wife, Royal Mother, Queen-In-Waiting

HARRY: Popstar Prince

One Direction: Your Backstage Pass To The Boys, The Band, And The 1D Phenomenon

* * *

Don't delay! Check them out today!

Made in the USA
Middletown, DE
22 March 2019